About the author: Dr Penny Stanway practised for several years as a GP and child-health doctor before becoming increasingly fascinated by researching and writing about healthy diets and other natural approaches to health and wellbeing. Penny has written more than 20 books on health, food and the connections between the two. She lives with her husband on a houseboat in the Thames.

This edition published in the UK and USA 2019 by
Nourish, an imprint of Watkins Media Limited
89–93 Shepperton Road, London N1 3DF
enquiries@nourishbooks.com

Design and typography copyright © Watkins Media Limited 2019

Text Copyright © Dr Penny Stanway 2019

Dr Penny Stanway has asserted her right under the Copyright, Designs
and Patents Act 1988 to be identified as the author of this work.

1 3 5 7 9 10 8 6 4 2

Managing Editor: Daniel Hurst
Editor: Amy Christian
Head of Design: Georgina Hewitt
Typeset by: Integra Software Services Pvt. Ltd, Pondicherry
Production: Uzma Taj

Printed and bound in Great Britain by TJ International Ltd.

A CIP record for this book is available from the British Library

ISBN: 978-1-848993-67-9

Note/Disclaimer: The material contained in this book is set out in good
faith for general guidance and no liability can be accepted for loss or expense
incurred in relying on the information given. In particular this book is not
intended to replace expert medical or psychiatric advice. This book is for
informational purposes only and is for your own personal use and guidance.
It is not intended to diagnose, treat, or act as a substitute for professional
medical advice. The author is not a medical practitioner nor a counsellor,
and professional advice should be sought if desired before embarking on any
health-related programme.

www.nourishbooks.com

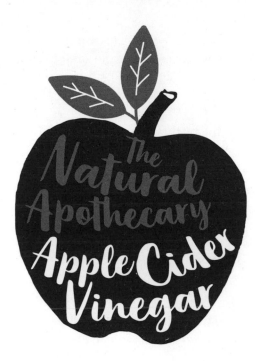

The
Natural
Apothecary

Apple Cider
Vinegar

DR PENNY
STANWAY

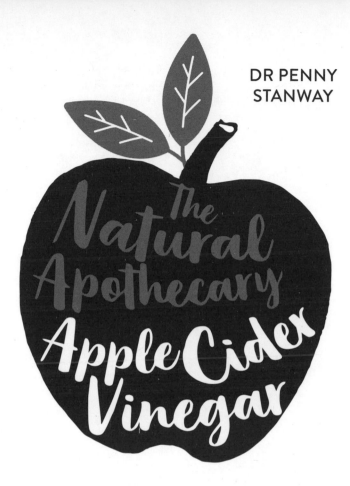

The
Natural
Apothecary
Apple *Cider*
Vinegar

USES FOR HOME, HEALTH
AND BEAUTY

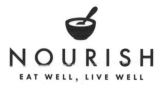

NOURISH
EAT WELL, LIVE WELL

CONTENTS

INTRODUCTION

For many thousands of years, people have been using natural products to soothe, treat, beautify and cleanse. Herbs and spices, vegetables, fruits, nuts and berries (as well as secondary products such as olive oil and vinegar) have been mixed together to create traditional remedies that have been passed down through the generations. Many of these ingredients are still used in commercial products today, although are now often combined with harsh chemicals.

Today, we are used to relying on pharmacies and supermarkets, where there are hundreds of available products, each with a different purpose. We apply creams and ointments for various aches and pains, take vitamin supplements, and spend a fortune on lotions and potions for our skin, nails and hair. The number of cleaning products that are now on offer can be quite overwhelming!

By going back to basics, and taking a more natural approach to how we treat our diets, health, beauty regimes and household management, we are taking back control of what we are putting into our bodies and what we are exposing our families to.

Apples are the most popular fruit in the world, and as the saying goes, 'an apple a day keeps the doctor away'.

Apples, apple juice, cider and cider vinegar have a long history and are much loved around the world, able to promote and protect our health and wellbeing. What's more, cider vinegar is a cheap and efficient source of help in the home.

Archaeologists believe that apple trees originated around the Caspian Sea and the Black Sea, and that people ate apples as far back as 6500 bc. Apple cultivation spread to Europe and in the 16th century King Henry VIII instructed his fruiterer to search the world for the best varieties, so he could set up orchards in England. Apple cultivation spread to the US, Australia, New Zealand, South Africa and South America. Nowadays, more than 7,500 varieties of apple are grown worldwide, and in many countries either home-grown or imported apples are available year-round.

Historians are unsure when people first enjoyed cider, but they know it was a common drink in Britain in the first century bc and think it was probably available around the Mediterranean in the 1st century ad. In contrast, archaeologists say that cider vinegar has been used for much longer, since traces of it exist in Egyptian urns dating from 3000 BC.

> The word 'vinegar' comes from the Old French 'vyn egre', which in turn came from the Latin 'vinum' + 'acer' ('wine' + 'sour').

A mild acid, that is relatively easy to produce, vinegar has a long history of use in industrial and medical spheres as well as in the home. Vinegar is a liquid primarily made up of acetic acid and water. It acts as corrosive agent and a preservative as well as being useful as a cleaning fluid. It is inexpensive and readily available, and homemade versions can be made relatively simply.

Vinegar is most often made from fruit or grains, or from alcoholic drinks, such as cider. Other types of vinegar include:

— fruit vinegars
— balsamic vinegar
— cane vinegar
— grain vinegar, such as rice vinegar or malt vinegar
— spirit vinegars, such as wine vinegars or sherry vinegar

Vinegar has traditionally been thought to offer many health benefits, and a surprising number of common ailments can be treated using cider vinegar, see pages 34–81.

Vinegar has antibacterial properties and can be used to cleanse and deodorize your body. Cider vinegar is a mild enough acid that is a helpful aid in maintaining the skin's natural acidity (see page 85).

Cider vinegar is also useful for many household chores and can help keep your home fresh, clean and sparkling. It also makes a great pest-controller! For environmentally-friendly, non-toxic ideas for using cider vinegar as a natural cleaning product, see pages 100–115.

NOTE

- What the English call 'apple juice' is known as 'cider' or 'sweet cider' in some countries, including the US.
- What the English call 'cider' is called 'hard cider' in some countries, including the US.

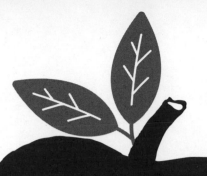

CHAPTER ONE

ABOUT CIDER VINEGAR

ABOUT CIDER VINEGAR

Making cider vinegar involves two basic types of fermentation. First, the sugars of apple juice are fermented to the alcohol of cider. Then the alcohol of cider is fermented to the acetic acid of cider vinegar (a process sometimes called 'acetification'). The colour of cider vinegar is a light brownish-yellow. It can be cloudy or clear. It can also be pasteurized (in which case it contains no microorganisms) or unpasteurized (in which case it contains some of the cloudy mass of fermentation bacteria called the 'vinegar mother').

Before we look at cider vinegar, let's go back to basics, and the fruit which it comes from. When you eat an apple, you aren't just getting a sugary source of 50 calories with some fibre and vitamin C. You are consuming a veritable treasure chest of health-promoting substances, some of which occur in such richness in only a few other foods. For example, apples are one of the most plentiful sources of pectin fibre and phenolic compounds such as quercetin. This explains why apples are the fruits most consistently associated with a reduced risk of certain chronic diseases, including heart disease, cancer, and diabetes, and why consuming apples, apple juice and cider vinegar really can make a difference to our health and wellbeing.

Apple juice

Apple juice is called 'apple cider' in the US and parts of
Canada. Apple juice diluted with water, or sweetened with
added sugar, must be labelled as an 'apple drink' or 'apple-
juice beverage'. Juicing apples requires mechanical pressing,
which produces cloudy juice.

Other possible processes include:

- Filtering of particulate material, including cellulose,
  pectins and proteins. This produces clear juice.
- Pasteurization, to prevent enzymes turning sugars to
  alcohols, and to protect against the growth of moulds
  and bacteria. This gives the juice a shelf life of up to two
  years. Unpasteurized juice should ideally be consumed as
  soon as possible.

The less processing there is, the smaller the loss of nutrients
and other valuable phytochemicals. Cloudy (unfiltered)
juice is slightly richer in fibre than is clear (filtered) juice.
It is also much richer in valuable phenolic compounds,
containing, for example, a much higher amount of
proanthocyanidins. And while it contains around half the
amount of phenolic compounds of apples themselves, clear
juice contains only up to a third or so.

Cider

Cider is an alcoholic beverage made by the fermentation
of apple juice. In the US, any fermented apple juice
containing more than 0.5 per cent ABV (alcohol by
volume, meaning millilitres of alcohol per 100 millilitres
of liquid) is called 'hard cider'. In the UK, 1.2 per cent

ABV cider is designated 'low-alcohol' cider. More often, the alcohol content of cider varies from less than 3 per cent ABV (for example, French *cidre doux*) to 8.5 per cent ABV or more (for example, in traditional English ciders). The flavour of ciders differs according to the apples or blends of apples used. Their colour varies from very pale gold ('white cider') to rich golden brown. The trend today is to make cider from a single crop of a single apple variety. The flavour of such a cider reflects the particular blend of volatile phytochemicals in that variety of apple; the cider can also be sold as being of a defined 'vintage'. You can use any apples to make cider; however, many cider makers like to include cider apples in their chosen blend. This is because these contain higher levels of tannins and more malic acid and other organic acids than do sweet 'dessert' apples, and give cider a characteristic 'bite'.

Cider apples are grouped in four categories according to their flavour components:

- Bittersweets are high in sugar, which raises the cider's alcohol content. They are also relatively high in tannins, so the cider is quite bitter.
- Bittersharps are high in tannins and fruit acids (for example, malic acid), so the cider is relatively bitter and sharp.
- Sweets are high in sugar, which raises the cider's alcohol. They are low in tannins and fruit acid, so the cider has little bitterness or sharpness.
- Sharps are high in acidity, which adds sharpness to their cider. They are low in sugar and tannins, so the cider is a little less alcoholic or bitter.

Cider's nutritional content relates to that of the apple juice from which it came, the type of fermentation, and any extra processing (such as filtration or pasteurization). Cloudy cider has a higher concentration of pectin and phenolic compounds than clear cider. For example, clear cider may have only 1–5 per cent of the proanthocyanidin content of cloudy cider. Cider contains relatively high levels of antioxidants: indeed, half a pint contains the same amount as a glass of red wine.

Lastly, cider contains fermentation products such as alcohol (derived from the apples' sugar) and small amounts of lactic acid (derived from the apples' malic acid, and which can add an interesting flavour). Cider is increasingly fashionable, but, however enjoyable it may be, it's wise to keep your alcohol intake within recommended limits.

To make cider, cloudy or clear apple juice is either left to ferment naturally, or wine yeast is added to speed fermentation and make it more reliable. Shortly before fermentation ceases, the cider is siphoned off, leaving a sediment of dead yeast cells and other material at the bottom of the container. This is called 'racking from the lees'. Sparkling cider is made by allowing fermentation of the remaining sugar and, perhaps, adding more.

Most commercially produced cider is also treated in other ways. It is usually pasteurized – heated to 71°C (160°F) or treated with ultraviolet light to kill bacteria and moulds.

Unpasteurized cider can be risky for pregnant women, young children and people with poor immunity. But while pasteurization renders cider safer and increases shelf life, it can slightly alter its flavour. It also destroys enzymes and inhibits oxidation, giving a less distinct flavour.

What's more, much commercial cider is made from apple concentrate, contains artificial colourings, sweeteners, preservatives and enzymes, and is filtered. It may have a source of nitrogen added and be stored under compressed carbon dioxide gas. All this makes cider production more reliable and changes the colour, clarity and flavour of cider in ways some people prefer. Others prefer the appearance and flavour of simply made 'natural' or 'real' cider.

Cider vinegar

Cider vinegar is not a rich source of nutrients. One tablespoon, for example, contains a little carbohydrate, very small amounts of minerals, extremely tiny amounts of trace elements, and virtually no protein, fat, vitamins or fibre. Some people claim it's a good source of calcium, but it isn't. We need around 1,000mg of calcium a day from food. One tablespoon of cider vinegar contains only 1mg, whereas one tablespoon of milk contains 20mg. There is a paradox here, though, because many people, including around one in two over-60s, make insufficient stomach acid for optimal absorption of calcium and certain other minerals. Cider vinegar can increase stomach acidity for such people, in which case it increases the absorption of calcium from foods.

Cider vinegar has many health-giving properties. Many come from its organic acids (such as acetic and lactic acids and, perhaps, traces of malic acid). These acids are mainly responsible for its antifungal, antibacterial and antiviral actions. Malic acid, the main organic acid in apple juice, is fermented to milder lactic acid during alcoholic and acetic fermentation. A by-product of this malolactic fermentation is a chemical with an attractive flavour that also contributes to the flavour of Chardonnay wine. Most commercial cider vinegars contain 5 per cent acetic acid.

Cider vinegar adds to the stomach's natural acidity. It is absorbed from the gut into the bloodstream and almost completely oxidized in the body's cells to produce energy. Although it contains acids, its overall effect, once absorbed from the gut, is usually said to be slightly alkaline. Certain scientists explain this by saying that if vinegar is burnt in the laboratory to a dry ash, this is alkaline when tested with a pH (acid-alkaline) meter. They say the oxidation of vinegar's acids in cells to produce energy is equivalent to vinegar being burnt in the laboratory.

Cider vinegar tablets are available, but may contain no cider vinegar at all! Instead they may contain weak organic acid salts and flavourings that make them smell vinegary.

Good cider vinegar is aged slowly. Its flavour is enriched and its composition made more complex during fermentation and subsequent ageing by volatile compounds such as aldehydes, ketones, alcohols, ethyl acetates, enzymes, phenolic compounds, salicylates and carboxylic acids (such as acetic, malic, lactic and succinic acids).

Buying cider vinegar

To gain most benefit from cider vinegar, it is recommended that you buy 'raw' organic vinegar, which is available from healthfood stores, larger grocery stores and online. Raw cider vinegar is unfiltered, unpasteurized, unprocessed and unheated. It is cloudy, rather than clear, and will often contain the 'mother'. It does not contain any artificial flavourings or chemicals.

VINEGAR MOTHER

This is a cloudy substance that sits at the bottom of a bottle of raw vinegar – it results from the fermentation process and contains most of the live bacteria and enzymes which make cider vinegar so good for us.

Making cider vinegar

Cider vinegar results from the fermentation by *acetobacter* bacteria of the sugar in cider to acetic acid. It's easier to make home-made cider vinegar than to make cider, because yeast is the only thing you'll need to add. The flavour of home-made cider vinegar is often more delicate and complex than that of the commercial sort, and because it has not been pasteurized, its flavour may continue developing over several years.

Most commercial producers convert cider to cider vinegar within a few hours by using a large fermenter with forced aeration and added *acetobacter*. Domestic cider-vinegar makers cannot buy these bacteria and most commercially produced vinegars do not work as a starter to set off and encourage fermentation, since they have been pasteurized and so contain no *acetobacter*. Wild *acetobacter* bacteria eventually find their way into cider, but adding an active starter (*see* below) aids fermentation. Use wooden, glass or food-grade stainless steel containers when making or storing cider vinegar. Do not use other metal, plastic, or glazed ceramic containers.

- Home-pressed apple juice and home-brewed cider and cider vinegar have distinctive flavours. Cloudy apple juice and cider contain tiny fragments of suspended apple pulp and because of this they are richer in pectin, phenolic acids and certain other health-promoting phytochemicals than are clear juice and cider.
- When making apple juice, cider or cider vinegar, choose containers made from food-grade stainless steel or plastic, or glass. Don't ever let cut-up or crushed apples, apple juice, or cider come into contact with containers, utensils or equipment containing iron, copper or lead.
- Very, very important – to avoid spoilage of juice, cider or cider vinegar by unwanted microorganisms – is to wash containers, utensils and equipment extremely thoroughly, using very hot water and no soap, then rinse well. Your kitchen and your hands should also be very clean.
- Some people recommend extra cleaning with a sulphite solution (for example, made by adding Campden tablets to water); they may also add this to their fermenting cider. However, quite a few people are sensitive to sulphites. Also, the amounts of sulphite usually do not actually sterilize – so they may leave some unwanted bacteria untouched.

To make cider vinegar at home, you will first need to make apple juice. The most important decision you'll need to make is which variety or varieties of apple to use, as this determines the proportions of sugar and acid that will be present in the juice. Dessert apples tend to be sweet. Cooking apples tend to be more acidic, or tart. Blending the two types – for example, ⅔ sweet apples to ⅓ tart apples – enables you to adjust the sweetness and acidity of the resulting juice. Cider apples are not suitable for making apple juice for drinking. Apples must be clean and have no trace of mould.

To make cloudy apple juice
As a rough guide, 9kg (20lb) of apples yields 4½ litres (1 gallon) of juice

---

SELECTING APPLES

Apples for making juice should be newly picked, firm and shiny and definitely unbruised, undamaged and rot-free. They can be of one variety, or several – three varieties, for example. Strongly flavoured dessert apples give a good flavour, especially if you add crab apples for a hint of bitterness from their high tannin content. Bittersweet and bittersharp varieties of cider apples have relatively high tannin levels too. The sweeter apples are, the more alcoholic their juice. Autumn-gathered apples tend to be sweeter than summer ones.

---

1 Wash the apples in cold water.
2 Either cut the apples into tiny pieces that are smaller than peas, or crush (pulp, grind or mince) them using a

food processor or a fruit mill or crusher (from a wine-makers' supplier). They could even be pulped by fitting a pulping attachment (a blade called a Pulpmaster) to an electric drill or crushed (very carefully) with a hammer.

TIP Crushed apple pulp is called pomace and rather than throw it away you can add it to cut-up whole apples to make apple pie.

3 Press the crushed or cut-up apples. Use an apple press (bought or hired from a wine-makers' supplier) to extract the juice from the milled apples by cold-pressing. Newly pressed apple juice goes brown within a few minutes, and it is this 'tanning' that is largely responsible for the final colour of the juice.

The apple juice can be drunk at once, or kept it in the fridge for 7–14 days (any longer and it will begin to ferment). The cloudiness may settle as sediment at the bottom of the bottle so, if necessary, stir or shake the juice before you drink it.

You can help prevent the natural browning of apple juice (caused by oxidation of its tannins) by adding 1g of powdered vitamin C (ascorbic acid, from a wine-makers' supplier) to each 2 litres (3½ pints) of freshly pressed juice.

Some people make large quantities of juice and preserve it by freezing, pasteurizing (which destroys some of its vitamin C), or chemical treatment. Preservation prevents microorgan- isms 'spoiling' (fermenting) the juice and thereby creating gases which build up pressure in capped bottles that could make them explode. Freezing is the best method for home-made apple juice.

Freezing

To freeze apple juice, pour it into plastic containers, filling them not quite full (to allow for expansion), then cover and freeze. Frozen juice keeps well for at least a year. Shake thawed juice before drinking it, as its valuable cloudiness tends to settle as sediment. Keep it in the fridge after thawing.

To make cider vinegar

1 Make apple juice as on pages 13–14, noting that the sweeter the apples, the stronger the cider vinegar will be.
2 Consider adding brewer's yeast (according to the instructions on the packet); while not essential, this hastens alcoholic fermentation.
3 Put the juice into an open container, filled only three-quarters full, to ensure easy entry of *acetobacter* bacteria, cover with a muslin cloth tied around the rim of the container to exclude insects, and leave in a warm dark place. It should start bubbling within a few days.
4 Aerate the mixture each day by stirring vigorously, and keep warm at around 18–30 °C (65–86 °F). Gradually a whitish gel-like raft of 'vinegar mother' will form. This contains *acetobacter* bacteria plus the cellulose they make to keep them floating, since they need plenty of air.
5 Consider speeding fermentation by adding some previously made unpasteurized and preservative-free cider vinegar. Not only do *acetobacter* thrive in a more acidic environment, but the added vinegar will probably supply some live *acetobacter* from remaining traces of vinegar mother, and these will act as a starter. Add about 100ml (just under 4fl oz) to each litre of fermenting liquid.

6 Leave the cider vinegar undisturbed for four weeks if you
   have added yeast, eight weeks if not, then taste it. If you
   think it is vinegary enough, siphon the rest into bottles,
   filling them to the top and capping them. If not vinegary
   enough, leave it for as long as it takes, tasting every week.
   It is better not to filter cider vinegar. And there is no
   need to pasteurize small quantities of home-made cider
   vinegar. Traces of vinegar mother may show as slight
   cloudiness or as gelatinous particles.

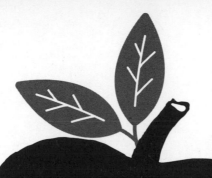

CHAPTER TWO

CIDER VINEGAR AND A HEALTHY DIET

2

CIDER VINEGAR AND A HEALTHY DIET

Some alternative therapists recommend drinking cider vinegar diluted in water every morning, as a daily health tonic. Try one or two tablespoons of vinegar in 250ml/1 cup water. Neat vinegar or anything stronger than this will be too acidic. The malic acid in vinegar is said to be beneficial to gut health. It also helps to break down carbohydrates, starches in particular, which can aid with bloating. It is said to make you feel fuller, preventing sugar cravings. For more on cider vinegar and health, see pages 34–81.

The saying, 'An apple a day keeps the doctor away', is proving very true. Fruit makes an invaluable contribution to good health. Researchers recommend at least five helpings of fruit and vegetables a day; two of every five can be fruit; and one of these two can be fruit juice. However, many people fail to get anywhere near five-a-day. A 2008 survey in the UK found that only 12 per cent of respondents had five-a-day, while 12 per cent had none.

Fruit is health-promoting and enjoyable, and apples are especially so. They are very rich in certain substances – for example, flavonoids and pectin – that have important health benefits. A 2004 research review found apples were more consistently associated with a reduced risk of cancer, diabetes and heart disease than any other fruit (or vegetable). Apple consumption was also linked with less asthma, better lung function and increased weight loss. While apple juice and cider are less rich in health-giving ingredients than apples, they have some value and are delicious to drink.

It make sense, then, to look at adding apples and their byproducts into your diet. Apples are brilliant on their own and a good complement to many other foods. Crisp dessert apples partner well with cheese, for example, and I suggest you experiment to see which varieties of apple you prefer with which types of cheese. You might start by trying a bronzy russet apple with a chunk of cheddar or nutty wensleydale, a sweet Red Delicious with a piece of Stilton or Dolcelatte, or a tart Granny Smith with some crumbly goat's cheese.

Apples are excellent in fruit salad and you can also add sliced, diced or shredded apple to vegetable salads – such as white, red or green cabbage salad, potato salad, beetroot salad, nut and celery salad and celeriac salad. Apple slices slowly dried in the oven, cooled, then stored in an airtight tin, are a great addition to picnics and lunchboxes. Apples can add a fragrant note to soup, and also form the base of many delicious sorts of chutney.

Cider isn't just a delicious beverage – it's great to cook with too. Substituting it for stock or water adds a fragrant and unusual note to casseroled meat, poultry or vegetables. Simmer cider in a saucepan until its volume has greatly reduced, then drizzle the resulting intensely flavoured liquid over plain yoghurt, or sweeten it as in the recipe for cider glaze, below. Cider makes a surprisingly attractive sorbet. And good mulled cider is the equal any day of good mulled wine.

Cider vinegar is most at home in the kitchen – use this fragrant tawny vinegar whenever a recipe specifies malt, wine or other vinegar. It's good, for example, for making salad dressings and many sauces – including mayonnaise, mint sauce, mustard and the South American chimichurri.

Sprinkle cider vinegar over fried fish and chips, or over soft herring roes that have been coated with flour then fried in butter and olive oil. And make gravy by adding a couple of tablespoons to the juices in the roasting pan in which you have cooked a joint of lamb.

Cider vinegar is a natural for pickling or marinating various vegetables and fruits. And it's an essential ingredient of many a savoury casserole.

The following recipes are quick and easy ways to add more cider vinegar into your diet.

CIDER VINEGAR INFUSIONS

Vinegar infusions are very easy to make and are a great way to use up fruits, especially berries, and herbs. Try raspberries, blackberries, thyme, rosemary, oregano, peppercorns, mustard seeds, garlic or chillies. Experiment with different flavours. Use the flavoured vinegars for dressing salads or vegetables.

1 Place your chosen ingredient in a sterilized glass jar, filling the jar about halfway, and chopping into small pieces if necessary.
2 Pour in enough cider vinegar to fill the jar.
3 Label the jar with the date and ingredients used.
4 Allow to infuse for at least two weeks, leaving the jar in a cool, dry place. Give the jar a gentle shake every few days.
5 Strain the vinegar into sterilized glass bottles, and label those as well.

Salad Dressing

This dressing makes lettuce leaves, other raw vegetables and other salad ingredients unusually enticing. You can vary it by adding herbs or spices.

6fl oz (180ml/¾ cup) olive, walnut or corn oil (or a mixture of any two)
2 tablespoons cider vinegar

2 teaspoons Dijon mustard
1 teaspoon clear honey
Black pepper

Put the ingredients in a bowl and whisk well with a fork.

Blender Mayonnaise

This home-made mayo is a real treat and is easily made in an electric goblet blender. If you find the flavour of olive oil too strong, use corn or sunflower oil instead.

2 tablespoons cider vinegar
1 egg
2 teaspoons Dijon mustard
1 teaspoon clear honey
black pepper

6fl oz (180ml/¾ cup) olive oil, or half and half olive and walnut oils
2 tablespoons just-boiled water (optional)

Put the cider vinegar, egg, mustard, honey and black pepper in the blender, and blend at high speed for a few seconds until smooth. Continue blending at a lower speed and very slowly pour in the olive oil (or olive and walnut oils).

Pickled onions

These are very simple to make and completely addictive. Serve them alongside cheeses, cold meats and other pickles, or as part of a traditional Ploughman's lunch.

70g (¼ cup) salt
325g (11½oz) shallots or small onions, peeled and trimmed
355ml (1½ cups) cider vinegar

1 teaspoon mustard seeds
½ teaspoon black peppercorns
1 bay leaf

1   Add the salt to 500ml (generous 2 cups) water in a large pan over a medium heat. Allow the salt to dissolve fully before removing from the heat.
2   Add the peeled onions to the pan and allow them to sit in the salty water overnight.
3   The next day, heat the vinegar, mustard seeds, peppercorns and bay leaf in a pan over a medium heat. Bring the mixture to a simmer, but do not allow to boil. Remove from the heat and allow to cool.
4   Drain the onions, rinse under cold water and dry them off with kitchen paper.
5   Place the onions in a sterilized jar, packing them in quite tightly. Pour over the cooled vinegar, with the spices, until the onions are covered.
6   Seal the jar and leave in a cool, dry place for at least four weeks until the onions are ready to eat. Once opened, keep refrigerated.

Bone Stock

This stock, made with a cooked chicken carcass, or with ham, pork, beef, lamb or fish bones, is very rich in calcium, due to cider vinegar releasing calcium from the bones. Use it as the basis of soup, or add it to casseroles or any other recipes that require stock.

cooked stripped chicken carcass, other meat bones, or fish bones

2 carrots, peeled and finely sliced

2 onions, peeled and chopped

2 cloves garlic, peeled and crushed or chopped

180ml (6fl oz/¾ cup) cider vinegar

1 teaspoon dried mixed herbs

black pepper

½ teaspoon salt

Put all the ingredients into a large saucepan and cover with water. Bring to the boil, cover and simmer for one hour, adding more water if necessary. Strain the stock into a bowl and use at once, or cool and freeze for another time.

Cucumber Pickle

This is brilliant with cold savoury food and a sure-fire hit whether served for solo repasts, family meals or festive gatherings.

2lb (900g) cucumber, peeled
and finely sliced
2lb (450g/3 cups) onions, finely
sliced
2 tablespoons salt
15fl oz (450ml, just under 2
cups) cider vinegar
12oz (350g/3½ cups) brown

sugar
½ teaspoon ground turmeric
½ teaspoon ground cloves
4 teaspoons mustard seed
4 teaspoons celery seed
(optional, but worthwhile if
you can get it)

1 Sterilize glass preserving jars, or jam jars with screw-on lids, by
   scalding with just-boiled water.
2 Put the cucumber, onions and salt into a bowl, mix well and
   leave for 3 hours. Rinse well in cold running water and drain in
   a sieve.
3 Put the cucumber and onions into a large saucepan, add
   the cider vinegar and bring to the boil. Simmer gently for 20
   minutes. Add the sugar, turmeric, cloves, mustard seed and
   celery seed and stir until the sugar has dissolved. Bring to the
   boil then simmer for 2 minutes.
4 Remove the cucumber and onions with a slotted spoon and
   put into the warm glass jars. Simmer the remaining syrup for
   15 minutes, then pour it over the cucumber and onions. Cover
   the jars tightly.

Beetroot and Horseradish Relish (Cwikla or Red Chrain)

This colourful accompaniment for fish, meat or cheese originated in eastern Europe and in Russia. Once you've tried it the odds are high you'll be a big fan.

1lb (500g) raw beetroot
2 tablespoons horseradish
   sauce
1 tablespoon wholegrain
   mustard

2fl oz (60ml, ¼ cup) cider
   vinegar
1 tablespoon sugar
plenty of black pepper

1   Boil the beetroots in their skins for 30 minutes or until tender when tested with a knife. Leave to cool, then rub off the skins and grate the beetroot.

2   Stir the horseradish sauce, mustard, cider vinegar, sugar and pepper into the grated beetroot.

Marinated Pears

Tickle your taste buds by eating these sweet-and-sour pears with cold meat, sausage or cheese.

2lb (1kg) hard pears, peeled, cored and quartered
water to cover
sugar
1 pint (550ml, 2½ cups) cider vinegar
1 pint (550ml, 2½ cups) water

1lb (450g, 2¼ cups) sugar
1 clove
pinch of cinnamon
bay leaf
1 teaspoon peppercorns
pinch of salt

1   Sterilize glass preserving jars, or jam jars with screw-on lids, by scalding with just-boiled water.
2   Cover the pears with water in a pan, bring to the boil and simmer for 15 minutes or until slightly soft. Drain and cool in the sieve under cold running water.
3   Put the vinegar, one pint of water, sugar, clove, cinnamon, bay leaf, peppercorns and salt into the pan, bring to the boil and simmer for five minutes. Gently add the pears, bring to the boil again, then cool. Put the pears into sterilized glass jars, fill with the liquid, then screw on the lids.

Tips for Cooks
Beans
Discourage flatulence by adding a tablespoon of cider vinegar to the water when soaking dried beans.

Cheese
Help prevent stored cheese hardening by wrapping it in muslin soaked in cider vinegar.

Eggs
- Poaching: put 2 teaspoons of cider vinegar in the water to help egg whites stay better formed.
- Hard-boiling: put 1 or 2 tablespoons of cider vinegar in the water to make eggs easier to shell.
- Boiling: put 2 tablespoons of cider vinegar in the water to help prevent shells cracking.

Jellies or jellied savoury dishes
Add a teaspoon of cider vinegar to the still-warm liquid to help the gelatine set.

Meat and fish
When marinating, braising, poaching or boiling meat, or poaching fish, add half a cup of cider vinegar to each cup of liquid to make the meat or fish more tender and to draw calcium from its bones.

Meringue
Add a teaspoon of cider vinegar to every 2 egg whites and leave to stand for 30 seconds before whipping. This increases their stiffness and makes meringues brilliantly white.

Pancakes
If you'd like to use buttermilk but you haven't any, add a tablespoon of cider vinegar to a cup of milk and leave it for five minutes before using.

Pastry
Instead of adding water to the flour-butter mixture, add flavour by adding cider vinegar, or half and half of cider vinegar and water.

Rice or pasta
Put a teaspoon of cider vinegar into the water and you'll find the cooked rice or pasta is less sticky.

Salads, vegetables and fruit
Washing with a cider vinegar solution may help remove certain pesticides and potentially harmful bacteria. To make the solution mix 1 part cider vinegar to 9 parts water, immerse the produce and let it soak for 5 minutes, then rinse well.

Soups, gravy or a savoury sauce
Add 2 tablespoons of cider vinegar to improve the flavour.

Stock made with a chicken carcass or other bones
Add a tablespoon of cider vinegar to the water to enrich the stock with calcium from the bones.

Vegetables
When boiling or steaming vegetables, add a splash of cider vinegar to the water while cooking to help the vegetables retain their colour.

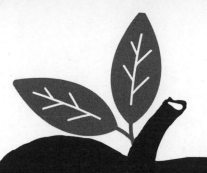

CHAPTER THREE

NATURAL REMEDIES FOR HEALTH

3

NATURAL REMEDIES FOR HEALTH

Reports of the healing properties of cider vinegar date from thousands of years ago. In 400 bc, the Greek doctor Hippocrates used it as an antibiotic and for general health. Samurai warriors used a vinegar tonic for strength, and a vinegar solution was used to prevent stomach upsets and treat pneumonia and scurvy in the US Civil War and to treat wounds in World War I.

There is no doubt that apples and apple juice are beneficial to our health. For more information on the specific ways that they can help with many common health problems, see pages 21–3. Traditional use, common sense and anecdotal evidence suggest cider vinegar can also help a wide variety of ailments, although few trials have been done. One reason is that it's difficult to get funding as cider vinegar can't be patented.

Cider vinegar is sometimes called a 'superfood'. These are foods that are thought to be nutritionally dense and therefore the best ones to include in our diets as part of a healthy lifestyle. Fruits such as blueberries or kiwi, nuts and seeds, beans and whole grains, leafy green vegetables and oily fish such as mackerel are often included in lists of the top superfoods that we should be eating, although the lists can be rather subjective.

In 1958 the term 'Honeygar' or 'Honegar' was coined by an American doctor writing about folk medicines. This refers to a mix of honey and vinegar and is available to buy today in pre-mixed bottles, clearly aimed at the health market. There are also several flavoured vinegar drinks ranges on the market. These often sold as detox products and include mixtures of cider vinegar with other superfood ingredients, such as pomegranate, goji berries or acai. If you find the taste of vinegar in water too strong, it might be worth trying these, although they may also contain high levels of sugar so always check the labels.

The list of ailments in this chapter details how and why cider vinegar can help, but don't forget that you can also discourage common ailments with a healthy diet (including a variety of superfoods), adequate hydration, regular exercise, daily outdoor light, effective stress management, a sensible alcohol intake and no smoking.

PLEASE NOTE

- The strategies outlined should not take the place of medical diagnosis and therapy.
- Anyone allergic to cider vinegar, apples or any apple constituent, such as pectin, should avoid them.
- The acidity of cider vinegar may temporarily soften tooth enamel, making it vulnerable to damage. So dilute it, use a straw, rinse your mouth with water afterwards, and don't clean your teeth immediately after.

- Excessive amounts of undiluted cider vinegar, or cider vinegar tablets, might damage the gullet and other parts of the digestive tract.
- Cider vinegar tablets may stick in the throat or gullet, so wash them down well.
- Prolonged use of cider vinegar could theoretically lower potassium, which could encourage toxicity from certain drugs (for example, digoxin, insulin, laxatives and certain diuretics).
- Cider vinegar affects blood sugar and insulin, so might
- have an additive effect if combined with diabetes medication.
- Cider vinegar may lower blood pressure, so it might have an additive effect if it is combined with high blood pressure medication.

Skin and hair

Acne

One cause of acne is overproduction of sebum due to over-sensitivity of sebaceous glands to testosterone. Other possibilities are changes in sebum and unusually sticky hair-follicle cells. Other triggers include the premenstrual fall in oestrogen, humidity, stress, certain drugs (for example, the progestogen-only pill), and polycystic ovary syndrome. A reduction in the skin's normal acidity may encourage infected spots.

Some people report that cider vinegar helps; if so, it could be because it kills bacteria, increases skin acidity, 'cuts' (emulsifies) skin oil, and reduces inflammation.

Regular treatment

Mix 1 part of cider vinegar with 4 parts of water. Apply with cotton wool, rinse after 10 minutes and repeat three times a day.

Corns and calluses

These are usually caused by ill-fitting footwear. Soaking the feet in a solution of cider vinegar is reputed to soften corns and calluses and hasten their demise.

Regular treatment

Add a cup of cider vinegar to a large bowl of warm water and soak your feet for 10 minutes a day. Afterwards, rub softened skin from the surface of the corn.

Eczema

Cider vinegar washes are a traditional remedy for eczema. The inflammation of eczema makes the skin's pH (acidity/alkalinity) rise above its normal slightly acidic pH range of 4.2–5.6. Normal acidity helps prevent infection in eczematous skin by inhibiting the multiplication of potentially harmful bacteria and fungi. Cider vinegar washes have nearly the same pH as normal skin.

Regular treatment

Try rinsing the affected area of skin with a mixture of equal volumes of cider vinegar and water twice a day. Avoid broken skin, as this will sting.

Warts

There are many anecdotal reports of cider vinegar curing warts. Some podiatrists use a more corrosive relative of acetic acid, dichloroacetic acid, to treat verrucas and other warts.

Regular treatment

Soak some cotton wool in cider vinegar and apply to the wart. Cover with a sticking plaster overnight. Repeat each night for 2 weeks.

Heat rash

Vinegar is said to soothe this itchy pimply rash.

Quick fix

Try applying a solution made by adding 1 tablespoon of cider vinegar to a cup of water.

Itching
Applying cider vinegar is said to help relieve itching.

Quick fixes
Try bathing in tepid bath water containing a cup of cider vinegar.

Or try applying neat cider vinegar to itchy skin, keeping it away from your eyes or other delicate parts.

Smelly feet
Cider vinegar soaks are said to reduce foot odour for some hours.

Quick fix
Soak your feet when necessary in a bowl of hot water plus a cup of cider vinegar.

Dandruff treatment

Dandruff is often associated with the fungus *Malassezia furfur*. Cider vinegar is a popular home remedy.

I cup cider vinegar   I cup warm water

1   Mix the cider vinegar and water together in a bowl.
2   Apply the solution to the scalp, rubbing it in with your fingertips.
3   Wrap your hair in a clean towel and wait for one hour before rinsing off the solution and then shampooing as normal.

Alternatively, massage neat cider vinegar into the scalp, cover with a towel and leave on for an hour. Repeat once or twice a week.

Age-related conditions

Ageing

Scientists have long searched for lifestyle factors that encourage long life and discourage age-related diseases (such as arthritis, heart disease, diabetes, cancer, osteoporosis and Alzheimer's). Long-lived peoples include certain groups in Russia (the Georgians), Pakistan (the Hunzas), Ecuador, China, Tibet and Peru. One link is that they tend to live at high altitudes; here, melting glacier water is rich in alkaline minerals such as calcium, which help the body maintain a healthy pH (acid-alkaline balance) without drawing calcium from the bones.

Apples, apple juice and cider vinegar have an alkalinizing effect in the body, so they, too, help conserve stored calcium.

Another possible factor encouraging these peoples' longevity is their consumption of fermented vegetables, fruit, milk, cereal grains, meat or fish. We don't yet know whether any benefit is caused by fermentation reducing the carbohydrate in the food; by any remaining fermentation bacteria; or by the presence of fermentation acids (such as lactic or acetic). Whatever the reason, folk medicine has long held that cider vinegar (fermented apple juice) helps protect against age-related disease; certainly, consuming it before a meal discourages high blood sugar afterwards (*see* Diabetes). Also, people with an age-related reduction in stomach acid (one in two over-60s in Westernized cultures) who take cider vinegar, aid their absorption of many nutrients (including protein, carbohydrates, fats, vitamins A, B, C and E, calcium, iron, magnesium, zinc, copper, chromium, selenium, manganese, vanadium, molybdenum, cobalt).

US researchers say mineral and vitamin deficiencies can accelerate the age-related decay of mitochondria (energy-providing structures in cells). Among the most important deficiencies are those of iron, zinc, biotin, pantothenic acid, magnesium and manganese.

Apples can help reduce inflammation associated with heart disease, arthritis and Alzheimer's, because they contain anti-oxidants and aspirin-like salicylates with anti-inflammatory actions. Unpeeled apples contain larger amounts. Apple juice contains smaller amounts.

Apple consumption is also associated with a reduced risk of cancer, strokes and type 2 diabetes.

Lastly, pectin binds to potentially toxic heavy metals such as aluminium and lead in the gut, which encourages their elimination. Indeed, pectin is regularly prescribed in Russia to remove heavy metals from the body. Such metals can form damaging 'cross-links' with brain and other cells. So, pectin's binding ability may mean it helps protect against premature degeneration and ageing.

Heal from the inside out
Until we know more, hedge your bets by eating an apple a day, and either adding cider vinegar to various recipes, or taking 2 teaspoons in a glass of water 2 or 3 times a day.

ALZHEIMER'S DISEASE

This results from brain-cell destruction and is associated with patches of amyloid protein and clusters of tangled nerve fibres. The cause isn't clear, but it can run in families and is more likely with age and after a serious head injury.

It's possible, though unproven, that eating apples might help prevent Alzheimer's or slow its development. One reason is that people with Alzheimer's tend to have high levels of the amino acid homocysteine, and are particularly likely to lack those B vitamins that help normalize homocysteine levels. Apples contain small amounts of folic acid and vitamin B6, which are among the B vitamins with the greatest effect. So they can make a useful contribution to the intake of vitamin B.

Several studies suggest that a small daily dose of aspirin or other non-steroidal anti-inflammatory drug discourages Alzheimer's. There isn't enough evidence for doctors to recommend taking such drugs long-term, and they can make the stomach bleed. But unpeeled apples, and apple juice, cider and cider vinegar made from unpeeled apples, are good sources of salicylates with aspirin-like qualities.

Arthritis

Inflammation links the many sorts of arthritis. Although some people claim that cider vinegar helps their arthritis, others say it doesn't. While it's certainly possible that people might react in different ways, there is no scientific evidence, so the jury remains out.

Apples could help reduce the inflammation that often accompanies arthritis, because they contain antioxidants (such as proanthocyanidin plant pigments, beta carotene, vitamin C, selenium) and aspirin-like salicylates.

Heal from the inside out
You may want to see if cider vinegar helps. Use it in salad dressings, soups or other recipes, or drink 2 teaspoons in a glass of water 3 times a day with meals.

Regular treatment
A folk remedy for arthritis in the hands or feet is to soak them 3 times a day in a solution made by adding 1 cup of cider vinegar to 3 cups of hot water.

Cataract
This clouding of the eye's lens affects many people over 65. Apples might discourage cataracts by helping protect against certain trigger factors, including diabetes, high blood pressure, smoking, infection and sunlight. Their eye-friendly nutrients include vitamins B2 and C, flavonoids and salicylates.

Cider vinegar is an unproven folk remedy for helping to prevent cataracts worsening.

Heal from the inside out
If you would like to try cider vinegar, add it to recipes or take 2 teaspoons in a glass of water 3 times a day for 6 months.

Osteoporosis
In this condition, affected bone is light and fragile and its cells are destroyed faster than they are created. Risk factors include age, too much or too little exercise, smoking, too little bright outdoor light, a lack of bone-friendly nutrients (calcium, magnesium, zinc, vitamins C, D and K and plant hormones), an early menopause, anorexia and various medications and illnesses (including gut and thyroid

disorders). Research increasingly points to inflammation and oxidation being involved.

Apples might help prevent osteoporosis or slow its development because of their antioxidants such as flavonoids, which counter inflammation and oxidation. Apples also contain the trace mineral boron, which researchers believe could improve oestrogen levels and reduce the loss of bone-friendly minerals in the urine. Another constituent, present in small amounts, is the phyto-oestrogen genistein. The rate of loss of bone density around the menopause is much lower in women with a high intake of plant oestrogens; apples contain only small amounts, nevertheless they might help as part of a healthy diet. Apple pectin is useful too, because good gut bacteria break this down, releasing short-chain fatty acids which raise acidity in the large intestine and thereby boost absorption of minerals such as calcium and magnesium.

Cider vinegar might be useful too. First, it renders calcium from food or in supplements more soluble and thus better absorbed. Second, it provides extra acidity in the stomach, which is useful for people in whom a lack of stomach acid causes poor absorption of calcium and certain other nutrients. Third, although vinegar is acidic, the net result of its digestion and metabolism is mildly alkaline.

Heal from the inside out
It's worth including apples and cider vinegar in your daily diet to help prevent or treat osteoporosis.

Memory loss
Anecdotal reports suggest that cider vinegar can aid memory.

Heal from the inside out

There's only very preliminary evidence that apples, apple juice and cider vinegar can improve memory or slow its loss, but nothing to be lost by including them in your diet.

Age spot lightener

The most common are brown freckles ('liver spots'), caused by normal ageing plus photo-ageing (accelerated ageing from sun exposure).
Some people report that applying cider vinegar – particularly if mixed with onion juice – lightens age spots.

1 onion   2 teaspoons cider vinegar

1   Peel and finely chop the onion, wrap it in a muslin cloth (cheesecloth), and squeeze to extract the juice into a small bowl.

2   Mix the cider vinegar with 1 teaspoon of the onion juice and apply the mixture to the freckles twice a day. They may begin to lighten within six weeks.

Digestion, diet and gut health

Anaemia
Iron-deficiency anaemia can be associated with low
stomach acid, which affects one in two over-60s. It can
also result from stress or the prolonged use of antacid or
acid-suppressant medication. A lack of stomach acid can
reduce iron absorption from food. Vitamin B12-deficiency
anaemia is another possible result of low stomach acid.

Eating apples could be particularly useful if you have
iron-deficiency anaemia. Gut bacteria break down apple
pectin, releasing short-chain fatty acids which raise acidity
and thereby boost iron absorption.

Heal from the inside out
If you have iron- or vitamin B12-deficiency anaemia, try
improving your absorption of either nutrient by drinking
a glass of water containing 2 teaspoons of cider vinegar
in water before each meal, or by adding cider vinegar to a
dressing for a first-course salad or soup.

Diarrhoea
Apple pectin is water-soluble and in the gut it forms a gel
that helps bind the bowel contents into stools and thereby
reduces bowel-opening frequency. What's more, 'good'
bacteria in the gut break down some of the pectin, forming
a protective coating for the gut lining which soothes any
irritation. This breakdown releases short-chain fatty acids
(such as butyric acid) with 'prebiotic' qualities, meaning
they nourish 'good' or 'probiotic' bowel bacteria such as
lactobacilli and bifidobac-teria. Pectin's prebiotic quality
makes colon cells stronger and better able to produce

protective mucus which helps prevent irritants sticking to and inflaming the gut lining.

Another type of apple fibre, cellulose, attracts water, bulks up bowel contents and makes them less runny. Cooking apples pre-softens their cellulose, helping it bulk up stools and reduce diarrhoea.

Cider vinegar can help kill diarrhoea-causing bacteria such as *Escherichia coli*, so it's useful for those people (such as one-in-two over-60s) with low production of stomach acid that would otherwise attack bacteria.

Heal from the inside out

If you have diarrhoea, try eating an apple every few hours. Raw apples are good, while cooking the apple first (for example, by stewing or baking it), pre-softens its cellulose, which may be useful if your bowel contents are rushing through very fast.

Regular treatment

You might also want to try drinking 2 tablespoons of cider vinegar in a glass of water 3 times a day.

Food intolerance

Poor production of stomach acid can occur with stress, prolonged use of antacids or acid suppressants and ageing.

Normal levels enable the digestive enzyme pepsin to break down proteins, but a shortage allows poorly digested protein to be absorbed into the blood and trigger allergy.

Heal from the inside out

If you think you might be short of stomach acid, try starting each main meal with a salad sprinkled with a cider vinegar and olive oil dressing, or first drink a glass of water containing 2 teaspoons of cider vinegar. Cider vinegar is considerably less acidic than stomach acid, but can nevertheless aid digestion.

Gallstones

Most gallstones contain cholesterol, others contain bile pigments or calcium salts. The bile often contains excess cholesterol and the gallbladder doesn't contract well. Such problems are more likely with obesity, constipation or diabetes, all of which may be helped by consuming apples and/or cider vinegar as part of a healthy diet.

The apple fibre pectin may bind and thereby help eliminate certain bile acids from the gut, which would prevent them being reabsorbed and used to make gallstones.

A tendency to gallstones may be linked with a lack of stomach acid, because this encourages the gallbladder to be inactive, which in turn encourages the formation of gallstones in the stagnant bile. A lack of stomach acid is more likely with ageing and stress and in people taking antacid or acid-suppressant medication.

Encourage gallbladder contractions with frequent meals that include something sour (such as cider vinegar) or bitter.

Heal from the inside out

If you suspect low levels of stomach acid, take 2 teaspoons of cider vinegar (added to a glass of water or a 'starter') before a meal, to increase stomach acidity. Cider vinegar's pH is 5, whereas stomach acid is more strongly acidic, with a pH of 1–2, but a little extra acid might be useful.

Gallbladder flush

Some people report success from a 'gallbladder flush'. This is said to soften stones and let them come out in the stools next day. Before trying a flush, discuss it with your doctor.

Days 1–6   Drink 1–2 litres of apple juice a day for 6 days.
Day 7   Miss supper; at 9pm, take 1–2 tablespoons of Epsom salts in a little water; at 10pm, drink 4 fluid ounces of olive oil shaken with 2 of lemon juice, then lie on your left side for 30 minutes before bedtime.

Peptic ulcer

Thick mucus normally protects the stomach and duodenum from stomach acid and the digestive enzyme pepsin. An ulcer can develop if something interferes with this mucus or with the lining cells or the volume of acid. The usual culprit is inflammation from infection with *Helicobacter pylori* bacteria. This is a major cause of stomach ulcers, stomach inflammation (gastritis) and stomach cancer. Around 2 in 5 of us are infected, though only 1 in 10 infected people develop an ulcer. Some people with ulcers make too much acid, but most don't, and some make too little.

It's theoretically possible that if someone with peptic ulcer symptoms tests positive for *H. pylori* and suspects a lack of stomach acid (for example, because acid-suppressants don't relieve symptoms), the acidity of cider vinegar might discourage the infection. But it might temporarily worsen ulcer pain.

Heal from the inside out

If you would like to try it, either drink a glass of water containing 2 teaspoons of cider vinegar each day, or use cider vinegar as a condiment or add it to recipes.

Indigestion and heartburn

Stewed apple is a favoured first food after a gastrointestinal infection. And organic acids in apples (for example, malic and tartaric) and cider vinegar (acetic acid) may help prevent indigestion caused by low stomach-acid production. Low stomach acid is encouraged by ageing, stress and prolonged use of antacids or acid-suppressant medication. Organic acids such as those in vinegar are weaker than gastric acid, but help provide an acidic environment for efficient protein digestion.

Heartburn is a frequent symptom of low stomach acid. Medical treatment is to suppress gastric acid with antacids, but this sometimes does no good or even worsens the problem. If antacids don't help, you may have low stomach acid. Consuming vinegar could then help by increasing your stomach acidity, though because its pH is only around 5, it cannot make the stomach as acidic as gastric acid (pH 1–2).

Heal from the inside out
To use cider vinegar to prevent problems, take 2 teaspoons in a glass of water before each meal, or add it to food.

If you have indigestion or heartburn, take 1 tablespoon in a glass of water. If it helps, the odds are that a lack of stomach acid was to blame.

Kidney stones
Cider vinegar is said to help dissolve common, calcium-containing stones. These are more likely when threatened overacidity of body fluids leads to calcium being withdrawn from bones and teeth and excreted in the urine to keep the body-fluid's pH (acid-alkaline balance) within its normal tightly controlled range. Cider vinegar, unlike other vinegars, is said to have a mild alkalinizing effect after it has been digested, so it might reduce the body's need to take calcium from bones. It might also help by reducing spikes of insulin in the blood after eating carbohydrate. Such foods otherwise raise insulin – a hormone that encourages stones by making the kidneys discharge more calcium in the urine.

Apples and apple juice may help prevent or dissolve stones, as they too have an alkalinizing effect. They also provide vitamin B6 and magnesium; this might help because, according to researchers, a lack of these nutrients encourages stones.

Heal from the inside out
Try including cider vinegar, apples and apple juice in your diet if you are prone to kidney stones.

Detox drinks

Store-bought cider vinegar detox drinks are available, but they can also be easily made at home. Combining cider vinegar with other health-promoting natural ingredients will allow you to harness all the benefits. Aim to drink one of these drinks every day. Add a little honey if you prefer your drinks to be sweeter.

Spicy lemon

1 tablespoon cider vinegar
1 tablespoon lemon juice
½ teaspoon cayenne pepper
½ teaspoon ground cinnamon

Add the ingredients to a cup of water and mix together well. Drink straight away.

Morning wake-up call

1 tablespoon cider vinegar
1 tablespoon lemon juice
¼ teaspoon turmeric

Add the ingredients to a cup of hot water, stir well to mix, and drink first thing in the morning to kick-start your metabolism.

Vitamin boost

2 tablespoons cider vinegar
¼ cup orange juice
¼ cup cranberry juice

Add the ingredients to a glass, taste, and dilute with as much water as required.

Antioxidant green tea

I cup green tea, made with leaves or a teabag	a few fresh mint leaves
	I tablespoon cider vinegar

Make a cup of green tea using leaves or a teabag. Add the mint leaves and stir the cider vinegar through. Allow to cool slightly before drinking.

Cider vinegar pills are sold at health food stores, pharmacies and online. The supplements, sold in tablet form, contain a dehydrated form of cider vinegar. There is little research available on the effectiveness of the pills, although they are said to have the same benefits on our health as ingesting cider vinegar in liquid form. Always check the ingredients on the label when buying supplements, as there may be other ingredients included. Drinking pure cider vinegar diluted with a little water is the safest way to ensure you are getting all the health benefits without any hidden 'nasties'.

Respiratory problems and allergies

Asthma

Inflammation and oversensitivity of airways causes wheezing, coughing and a tight chest. Possible triggers include cold air, exercise, certain foods, hormone changes, laughter, infection, various fumes, a sudden fall in air pressure, thunderstorms, allergy, and breathing too fast.

Apples and apple juice have an anti-asthma effect that seems stronger than that of any other food. This may result from their high levels of antioxidants such as quercetin, as these have a provable anti-inflammatory effect.

As for cider vinegar, Dr DC Jarvis, who studied 24 people in the US over two years in the 1950s, found their urine pH became highly alkaline before and early on in an asthma attack (*Folk Medicine*). On following his suggestion to drink cider vinegar, their urine rapidly returned to its normal acid pH and the asthma attack was less severe. He attributed this to its organic acids and potassium content.

Taking cider vinegar can restore some acidity to the stomach in someone with low levels of their own stomach acid. If you suspect this (for example, because you get indigestion that is not relieved by antacid medication), you might want to try taking cider vinegar either regularly each day to help prevent asthma, or early in an attack to help cure it.

Heal from the inside out

For an adult, put 1 tablespoon of cider vinegar into a glass of water and sip over half an hour. Wait another half-hour then repeat. Or put 1 tablespoon of cider vinegar in soup or salad dressing. For children, use less cider vinegar, depending on their size.

Hay fever
Cider vinegar is a traditional remedy for allergic rhinitis.

Heal from the inside out
Put a tablespoon of cider vinegar into a glass of water and sip the mixture over half an hour. Wait half an hour then repeat. Alternatively, add a tablespoon of cider vinegar to soup or other food.

First aid and infections

Bruises
These are associated with leaking of blood from tiny blood vessels. Applying a solution of cider vinegar to bruises is a folk remedy that could be worth trying to limit bruising and speed recovery.

Quick fix
Use a cotton pad to apply a solution of 2 tablespoons of cider vinegar in a cup of cool water.

Cold sores
These lip sores are caused by reactivation of a *Herpes simplex* viral infection by such triggers as stress, periods, infection, skin damage, sunshine and fatigue. Cider vinegar is an old home-remedy for this condition.

Quick fix
Try dabbing neat cider vinegar on your lip 3 times a day with a paper tissue or clean cotton pad if you think a sore is imminent.

You could also apply neat cider vinegar to an actual sore, but it might sting.

Ear infection
Cider vinegar is a traditional treatment for infection in the outer ear.

Regular treatment
Add 2 teaspoons of cider vinegar to an egg cup of water and apply with a cotton bud 3 times a day.

Fainting
Simple faints, or the dizziness that warns of them, are often associated with low blood sugar. Eating apples helps prevent this, mainly thanks to their content of the soluble fibre pectin, which helps keep the blood sugar steady by slowing the absorption of sugar from the gut.

Cider vinegar may help too, by slowing the rise in blood sugar after a meal; whether this is due to its acetic acid content or some other constituent is unclear.

Cider vinegar may also help prevent faints in those people – such as one in two over-60s – who have poor digestion caused by low stomach acidity, and who are also 'fast oxidizers' of sugar, meaning they feel hungry sooner after a meal than do most people. This is because its extra acidity improves protein digestion, so they can readily produce energy from protein when they have used up their available sugar.

Regular treatment
Eat apples as between-meal snacks, to help maintain normal blood sugar. Include cider vinegar in your main meals.

Sprains
Cider vinegar is said to relieve pain from a sprain, though why is unclear.

Quick fixes
Apply a cider vinegar compress to the affected area – for example, a face flannel squeezed out in a bowl of hot water plus a cup of cider vinegar.

Stings
Applying cider vinegar is a traditional way of treating a wasp sting. A bee sting requires baking soda (bicarbonate of soda) instead. An easy way to remember is 'V' for 'vasp' stings and vinegar, 'B' for baking/bicarbonate and bee stings. One possible mechanism is that it can convert certain toxins in wasp venom to less toxic acetate compounds.

Dousing with vinegar is a folk remedy for most jellyfish stings as it deactivates venom cells. But immersing the stung part in hot water, if available, for four minutes, is even more effective. Don't put vinegar on a sting from a Portuguese man-of-war jellyfish, though, since researchers say this could make the venom cells that are embedded in the skin discharge more venom.

Quick fix
Apply neat cider vinegar to a wasp or jellyfish sting, using a cotton pad.

Nosebleed
There are isolated reports that cider vinegar helps stem a nosebleed. Also, consuming cider vinegar is a traditional remedy for frequent nosebleeds

Quick fix

To see if cider vinegar helps stop a nosebleed, soak a cotton-wool ball in cider vinegar, lean your head backwards, then put the cotton-wool ball in the affected nostril.

Regular treatment

If you suffer from frequent nosebleeds, try drinking 2 teaspoons of cider vinegar in a glass of water 3 times a day for, say, 3 months.

Athlete's foot treatment

This fungal infection makes the skin between the toes sore and soggy, and is often picked up in changing rooms or around swimming pools. Anecdotal reports suggest cider vinegar might help.

4 tablespoons cider vinegar   10 drops tea tree oil

1   Fill a large bowl with warm water.
2   Add the cider vinegar and tea tree oil and mix well.
3   Bathe your feet in the water for 5–10 minutes every day to treat an outbreak of athlete's foot.

Head lice treatment

Cider vinegar does not kill lice effectively but can loosen the glue that sticks louse eggs (nits) to hairs.

250ml/1 cup cider vinegar
silicone-based conditioner (such as Pantene)

1   Add a cup of cider vinegar to a cup of water.
2   Apply to dry hair then leave for half an hour.
3   Wet the hair with water and smooth in lots of the silicone-based conditioner.
4   Comb the hair with a wide-toothed comb, then a fine-toothed one to remove any lice.
5   Now shampoo. Some nits may stay stuck to hairs, so do this wet-combing twice weekly for 2 weeks to catch newly hatched lice.

Coughs and colds

Colds and sore throat

Chewing an apple makes its pectin swell with water and form a soothing and protective layer of gel on an inflamed throat. This explains its use in certain commercial throat lozenges. An apple's vitamin C might shorten the length of a cold. Another benefit of apples is that fermentation of the pectin in the large intestine releases short-chain fatty acids (such as butyric acid) with 'prebiotic' qualities – meaning they nourish 'good' or 'probiotic' bowel bacteria, such as lactobacilli and bifidobacteria. These, in turn, have beneficial effects on the body's immunity.

A traditional remedy for a sore throat is to gargle with dilute cider vinegar; why this might help is unclear, though cider vinegar does have some antibacterial properties.

Quick fix

Put 1 tablespoon of cider vinegar in a glass of water and sip the mixture over half an hour. Wait half an hour then repeat the treatment. If you dislike cider vinegar in water, add it to soup instead.

Regular treatment

Gargle twice a day with a mixture made by putting 1 teaspoon of cider vinegar in a glass of water.

Cough

Vinegar has been used for millennia to fight infections; Hippocrates (460–377 BC), for example, prescribed it for persistent coughs. Apples, too, may help.

Traditional remedies for a cough involve applying some cider vinegar to the chest or pillow at night. By doing this small amounts of organic acid vapour from the vinegar might be absorbed into the body through the nose or skin, but why this might help remains unclear.

Quick fixes
Soak some brown wrapping-paper in cider vinegar and put it on your chest. Cover it with a towel, and relax for 20 minutes.

Alternatively, try sprinkling a little cider vinegar on to your pillow (covered with an old pillowslip!) each night.

General Health

Heavy periods
It's claimed that cider vinegar can ease heavy periods.

Regular treatment
If you would like to try this unproven home remedy, drink 2 teaspoons of cider vinegar in a glass of water 2 or 3 times a day, or add cider vinegar to your food.

Varicose veins
Cider vinegar is a traditional remedy for aching varicose veins, though why it might work is not clear.

Regular treatment
Dampen a small towel with cider vinegar and wrap it over troublesome veins twice a day, for half an hour each time.

Heal from the inside out
Either drink a glass of water containing 2 teaspoons of cider vinegar 3 times a day, or use cider vinegar as a condiment or in recipes.

Fatigue
Apples supply sugar plus small amounts of B vitamins that may help prevent or treat fatigue. More importantly, they supply fibre, which helps keep blood sugar steady, so helping prevent the low-blood-sugar swings sometimes associated with fatigue.

Theoretically, at least, cider vinegar could help tiredness associated with a lack of sufficient stomach acid. This prevents proper absorption of nutrients and is more likely with ageing and stress.

Heal from the inside out
See if it helps to eat an apple a day, and to take 2 teaspoons of cider vinegar 3 times a day, as a condiment, in a glass of water, or added to recipes.

Cramp
Possible triggers include insufficient dietary calcium, magnesium, potassium and vitamins B and C. These are all present in apples, so an apple a day might help.

Cider vinegar is a folk remedy for cramp, possibly because its acidity in the stomach improves calcium and magnesium absorption in the many people who produce sub-optimal levels of their own stomach acid.

Heal from the inside out
Include cider vinegar in recipes or take 2 teaspoons in a glass of water 3 times a day.

Quick fix
Mix 2 tablespoons of vinegar in a cup of warm water, soak a face flannel in this mixture, then put the flannel over the muscle and cover it with a thick towel.

Headache
Vinegar is a traditional remedy for a headache and familiar from the 'Jack and Jill' nursery rhyme in which Jack mends his head with 'vinegar and brown paper'. Why vinegar should help isn't clear, but some complementary practitioners believe headaches can result from various body 'buffer systems' having to work extra hard to keep the blood's pH (acid-alkaline balance) within its normal tightly controlled range; others believe headaches can result from this pH being at the alkaline end of normal. They recommend various remedies:

Quick fixes
Sponge the head with cider vinegar, or apply a flannel soaked in a pint (600ml) of water containing 2 tablespoons of cider vinegar.

Inhale organic-acid vapour by putting a tablespoon of cider vinegar into a vaporizer and staying near for, say, 15 minutes.

Regular treatment
Drink a cup of hot water containing 3 teaspoons of cider vinegar 3 times a day.

Hiccups
Possible causes are an overfull stomach, due to eating too much; low stomach acid slowing protein digestion; or fatty, sugary food slowing stomach emptying and encouraging fermentation. Cider vinegar is a traditional remedy.

Heal from the inside out

To try preventing frequent attacks, add cider vinegar to your food, or drink a teaspoon of cider vinegar in a glass of water before a meal.

Quick fixes

To try stopping hiccups, very slowly sip the same solution or swallow a teaspoon of neat cider vinegar.

Overweight and obesity

Apples contain the soluble fibre, pectin, which slows the absorption of sugar from the gut. This helps prevent hunger and overeating. Pectin can also interfere with the absorption of fat. One theory is that this is because pectins form a gel in the stomach, which mops up triglyceride fats and stops them being absorbed.

Vinegar has been said for thousands of years to promote weight loss. Early research suggests that if cider vinegar does indeed help, it does so by aiding satiety after eating, by helping the body burn calories faster and by helping compensate for any lack of stomach acid.

Low acidity in the stomach affects around one in two over-60s, and is encouraged by stress and prolonged use of antacid or acid-suppressant medication. Research associates low stomach acidity with poor absorption of many nutrients (including protein, vitamins B and C, calcium, iron, magnesium, zinc, copper, chromium, selenium, manganese, vanadium, molybdenum and cobalt). It also indicates that poor nutrient absorption can make people want to eat even when they are not hungry. Cider vinegar improves absorption of these nutrients by increasing stomach acidity. And by improving protein digestion, it may specifically help people who are 'fast oxidizers' of sugar and tend to feel very hungry within three hours or so of a meal. This is because they can readily produce energy from protein when they have used up their available sugar.

Cider vinegar also aids absorption of fats and vitamins A and E by stimulating the release of bile and pancreatic enzymes into the gut. It also slows the rise in blood sugar after a meal. This not only helps prevent high blood sugar, but also the low-blood-sugar swing that sometimes follows, and which can trigger desire to overeat. Whether its blood-sugar-lowering ability is due to its acetic acid or another constituent is unclear.

Heal from the inside out
It's worth including apples and cider vinegar in your diet if you would like to maintain or achieve a healthy weight.

Long-term/serious conditions

Diabetes and pre-diabetes

Cider vinegar and apples are proving useful in helping prevent or treat the high blood sugar of pre-diabetes and diabetes. This is important because high blood sugar encourages complications such as disease of the heart, eye and kidney.

Several studies suggest that vinegar may aid blood-sugar control in people with diabetes, and slow the progression of pre-diabetes to diabetes. One possible explanation is delayed stomach emptying. Another, courtesy of Japanese researchers is that acetic acid inactivates intestinal enzymes (disaccharidases) that convert sugars to glucose. This would help prevent blood sugar rising too high or too quickly, so lowering the need for insulin. Other studies suggest that acetic acid helps normalize the release of sugar from the liver, and the production of sugar in the liver from non-carbohydrate sources.

Other studies show that other acidic foods, including lemon juice, yoghurt, traditionally made slowly fermented bread, and kenkey (fermented corn) also reduce expected blood-sugar spikes after meals; some foods even being as powerful as the oral diabetes drug metformin. Frequent consumption of acidic foods is traditional in many countries and may help explain national differences in diabetes rates. Many such foods contain acetic acid, including Japanese sunomono (vinegar-treated vegetables), sumeshi (vinegared rice), potato salad, mustard, vinegared fish and chips, and vinegar-based dressings.

Heal from the inside out
It seems sensible for people with pre-diabetes or diabetes to eat an apple a day and either add cider vinegar to their food (or drink 2 teaspoons of cider vinegar in a glass of water 3 times a day, with meals), or eat other fermented foods or pickled products containing vinegar.

Strokes
A stroke ('brain attack') usually results from a blood clot interrupting the blood flow in one of the brain's blood vessels (thrombotic stroke). Less often it is caused by bleeding in the brain from an unhealthy artery (haemorrhagic stroke).

The main culprit behind a thrombotic stroke is the narrowing of an artery by atheroma. This fatty substance contains low-density lipoprotein cholesterol, which is readily oxidized by free radicals, making arteries inflamed, scarred and rough inside. Clots form on roughened artery walls, especially if blood is abnormally sticky. Risk factors include smoking, stress, unhealthy diet, obesity, high blood pressure, diabetes and chronic infections.

Preliminary evidence suggests that apples and cider vinegar help prevent high blood pressure, obesity and diabetes, so it's worth adding them to your diet.

Heal from the inside out
Include apples and cider vinegar in your daily diet.

High blood pressure
Risk factors include obesity, overactivity of the kidney hormone renin, insulin resistance (pre-diabetes), salt

sensitivity, age and genetics, though most often there is no obvious cause. Vinegar can affect several of these factors and preliminary studies suggest it can lower blood pressure.

There are five possible reasons. First, it increases nitric oxide (which relaxes blood vessels). Second, it acts like ACE-inhibitor blood-pressure medication (meaning it inhibits angiotensin-converting enzyme, thereby decreasing production of the blood-vessel constricting hormone angiotensin II). Third, it adds flavour, which helps salt-sensitive people reduce their salt intake. Fourth, adding it to casseroles or stocks containing meat bones releases some of their calcium; this could help the many people who have a low calcium intake, because calcium helps keep blood pressure healthy. Fifth, vinegar could lower blood pressure by encouraging weight loss.

Heal from the inside out
If you would like to try cider vinegar, add it to your food 2 or 3 meals a day, or take a teaspoon in a glass of water 3 times a day.

An apple a day
Some of the goodness from apples can be found in cider vinegar, but in addition, eating an apple a day will benefit your general health and might help prevent certain long-term illnesses. Eat apples unpeeled to get larger amounts of natural anti-inflammatories. Apple juice contains smaller amounts and the best choice is cloudy juice made from crushed whole apples. See pages 13–14 for a recipe for home-made apple juice.

Alzheimer's

It's possible, though unproven, that eating apples might help prevent Alzheimer's or slow its development. One reason is that people with Alzheimer's tend to have high levels of the amino acid homocysteine, and are particularly likely to lack those B vitamins that help normalize homocysteine levels. Apples contain small amounts of folic acid and vitamin B6, which are among the B vitamins with the greatest effect. So they can make a useful contribution to the intake of vitamin B.

Bronchitis and emphysema

These two types of chronic obstructive lung disease often require ever more intensive treatment. Studies suggest apples may help. Most researchers believe that antioxidants are protective, and some think the flavonol quercetin plays a key role. Other constituents that may help include other flavonoids, pectins and malic acid.

Cancer

Cancer results from mutation of a cell's DNA which allows the cell to continue multiplying instead of dying due to apoptosis (cell suicide) at its allotted time. Such malignant cells arise repeatedly during ordinary everyday life; most are destroyed by the immune system but a few grow into a cancer. Dietary factors that encourage certain cancers include a lack of anti-oxidants such as the flavonoid quercetin, as these normally mop up the free radicals (overactive oxygen particles) that are continually produced in the body and can damage cells. Several studies suggest that apples have anti-cancer properties and that their antioxidants are partly responsible. Other point to other apple phytochemicals, including pectins, pectin-like rhamnogalacturonans, and triterpenoids. Certainly pectin is broken down by gut bacteria, releasing short-chain fatty acids which raise acidity in the large intestine and thereby encourage apoptosis in colon cancer cells. What's more, experiments indicate that pectins and pectin-like rhamnogalacturonans have pronounced antimutagenic effects. Some alternative practitioners believe that diet can influence cancer by changing the body's pH (acid-alkaline) balance. Certainly a cancer itself can be relatively more acidic than normal tissue. But there is currently no scientific evidence to support their view.

Constipation
An unhealthy diet and dehydration are among the most likely causes of constipation. Eating unpeeled raw apples may help, because they are rich in water-soluble types of fibre called pectin and pectin-like compounds. Pectin dissolves in water to form a gel that makes stools softer and easier to pass through and from the bowel. Unpeeled apples also contain cellulose; this insoluble fibre attracts water, which makes stools softer, bulkier and easier to pass, and reduces their 'transit time' through the large intestine. Cloudy apple juice contains smaller amounts of pectin which may nonetheless be useful.

Gum disease
Chewing an apple boosts gum health, because repeated jaw movement increases the circulation of blood to the gums, and apples contain phenolic compounds called tannins which, studies suggest, help prevent periodontal (gum) disease.

Heart disease

Coronary heart disease encourages angina and heart attacks. Fatty atheroma collects in coronary artery walls and, when overly thick, the heart muscle no longer gets enough blood to enable it to pump properly. Free radicals in blood oxidize LDL (low-density lipoprotein) cholesterol in atheroma, producing oxidized LDL cholesterol – the dangerous sort. Free radicals are overactive oxygen particles and are encouraged by a poor diet, infection, smoking and stress. They also trigger immune cells to inflame artery walls. Atheroma and inflammation scar and roughen the lining of arteries, which encourages high blood pressure by making arteries less elastic; they also encourage blood clots that can block an artery and cause a heart attack.

Studies suggest that apples and apple juice help protect against heart disease, possibly thanks to their flavonoids such as quercetin and catechins.

Another possibility is that aspirin-like salicylates in apple peel may, like aspirin (acetyl salicylic acid), discourage heart attacks associated with inflammation of coronary arteries.

Finally, 'good' microorganisms degrade the apple fibre pectin in the large intestine, freeing useful short-chain fatty acids such as butyric acid. These acids reduce LDL cholesterol (the potentially dangerous sort) and increase HDL cholesterol (the potentially protective sort). They also inhibit C-reactive protein, a blood marker for inflammation and a predictor of cardiovascular disease.

High cholesterol

Apples can help prevent high cholesterol. People with an unhealthy balance of LDL (low-density lipoprotein) and HDL (high-density lipoprotein) cholesterol, tend to develop a cholesterol-rich layer of atheroma in their arteries. This impairs their circulation. Also, the presence of oxidized LDL cholesterol in atheroma stiffens arteries and encourages high blood pressure, heart attacks and strokes.

Pectin in apples, and to a lesser extent in cloudy apple juice, absorbs cholesterol and triglycerides in the gut and eliminates them from the body. One way it does this is by increasing the viscosity of the contents of the small intestine, which reduces the absorption of cholesterol from food or bile. Another is that 'good' microorganisms degrade pectin in the large intestine, liberating short-chain fatty acids (such as butyric acid) which inhibit cholesterol absorption, suppress cholesterol production in the liver, and boost HDL cholesterol.

Studies using whole apples show that a combination of pectin and vitamin C lowers cholesterol more than does pectin alone; and the combination of pectin and phenols lowers cholesterol and triglycerides more than either alone. The decreases are small but worthwhile. Eating one large apple a day lowers cholesterol by up to 11 per cent. Eating two lowers cholesterol by up to 16 per cent. The cholesterol lowering effect of four a day can equal that of a statin drug!

Some alternative practitioners explain that cholesterol is an acidic by-product of fat metabolism. They say a healthy diet containing plenty of alkaline-forming foods (such as apples and cider vinegar) makes the body better able to prevent atheroma accumulating in the arteries, and to dissolve or neutralize and then eliminate cholesterol.

Irritable bowel syndrome (IBS)

Possible symptoms include pain, constipation, diarrhoea, passing mucus, bowels never feeling empty, wind and bloating. One in three people sometimes have an irritable bowel; one in five of these have frequent trouble – which is then called irritable bowel syndrome (IBS). Apples' soluble pectin fibre may reduce symptoms, partly because it makes stools softer and easier to pass.

Low immunity

Apples may boost immunity. First, their vitamin C is useful for immunity. Second, their pectin fibre is degraded by 'good' microorganisms in the large intestine, liberating short-chain fatty acids such as butyric acid. These aid immunity by stimulating production in the spleen of helper T cells, antibodies, white blood cells and cytokines. They also inhibit C-reactive protein, a blood marker of inflammation.

Parkinson's disease

This results from degeneration of brain cells that produce the neurotransmitter (nerve-message carrier) dopamine. There's usually no apparent cause but scientists believe genes and brain infection can play a part. Studies suggest an apple a day helps reduce the risk of neurodegenerative disorders such as Parkinson's.

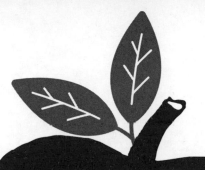

CHAPTER FOUR

NATURAL
BEAUTY
TREATMENTS

4

NATURAL BEAUTY TREATMENTS

Cider vinegar (and apples) are not only valuable for our health but also have a rightful place in the beauty parlour. The main reason that cider vinegar is such a popular beauty aid is that its organic acid concentration of about 5 per cent helps maintain the skin's natural acidity. Most other vinegars – except, for example, naturally fermented wine vinegar – are more acidic than this and therefore unsuitable for skin care.

Normal skin has a slightly acidic surface layer called the 'acid mantle' or hydro-lipid film. This contains:

- The fatty acids of skin oil (sebum)
- Lactic acid and various amino acids from sweat
- Amino acids and pyrrolidine carboxylic acid from 'cornifying' (hardening) skin cells.

The skin's acid mantle has a pH (acid/alkaline balance) of 4.5–5.75 over most of the body. (A 'neutral pH is 7; below this is acidic, above is alkaline). The pH of the skin in the armpits and around the genitals is around 6.5, which is less acidic. Normal skin pH tends to be slightly more acidic in men than in women.

Apples contain many nutrients that are a boost for healthy skin. Most importantly, they contain vitamin C, which helps to build collagen in the skin, preventing fine lines and wrinkles, and is also an antioxidant so can help your skin fight damage to your skins cells that might have been caused by over-exposure to the sun or to pollution.

Normal acidity helps activate the enzymes that enable the production of the lipids (oily fats) present in the skin's hydrolipid film. It also encourages skin to repair itself after mechanical or chemical damage. All this is important, because intact healthy skin is relatively impermeable. This means that water is much less able to escape through the skin (other than via perspiration), and potentially harmful substances and microorganisms are less able to get in. Normal skin acidity also encourages a normal skin flora – the typical populations of various bacteria and fungi that inhabit healthy skin. A normal skin flora helps prevent potentially harmful microorganisms from multiplying and causing infections.

Any loss of normal skin acidity encourages drying, cracking and itching. What's more, eczema or other inflammation tends to make skin more alkaline. Washing with most types of soap increases this alkalinity and makes the skin even more vulnerable to irritation and infection.

Cider vinegar has become very fashionable in beauty circles. There are now many commercially-made products available on the market which claim to harness the benefits of cider vinegar. Many of these products contain other natural ingredients, and can be a convenient way to introduce cider vinegar into your beauty regime, but make sure that you check the product labels for any added 'nasties'.

Most soaps, even 'mild' soaps, glycerine soaps, 'baby soaps' and 'beauty bars', have an alkaline pH of 7–9. Washing with such soap destroys the skin's protective acid mantle. Healthy, unbroken skin can recover from this increase in pH but the restoration of normal acidity takes time – generally between half an hour and two hours or more; and twice-daily washing with alkaline soap slightly reduces the restored acidity level. Certain soaps are even more alkaline, with a pH of 9.5–11, so they compromise skin acidity even more. The pH of Dove soap is 6.5-7.5, which is relatively low for a bar soap. Only a very few bar soaps have a pH similar to that of normal skin.

However, the pH of many liquid soaps, non-soap cleansers and bath and shower gels is closer to that of normal skin; and a few, for example, Johnsons pH 5.5 Hand Wash, have a pH similar to that of normal skin. Using a home-made skin cleanser containing cider vinegar avoids the loss of normal acidity that accompanies washing with most types of soap. Another idea, if you want to continue using alkaline soap, is to rinse your skin afterwards with a home-made skin splash containing cider vinegar, so as to restore the skin's normal acidity.

Cider vinegar can also restore acidity to hair that has been washed with an alkaline shampoo. Most shampoos are alkaline and can leave newly washed hair dull and lacklustre. They also temporarily destroy the normal acidity of the scalp, leaving it more prone to dryness, irritation and infection. However, a cider vinegar rinse can make the hair shinier than it would otherwise be. It can also enhance natural highlights in hair.

Because of its antibacterial properties, cider vinegar also has deodorizing properties that are particularly useful for armpits and feet.

NOTE

Always test out home-made beauty treatments on a small patch of skin before using.

Bathroom hero

Keep a bottle of cider vinegar to hand in your bathroom cabinet – it can be used for a variety of everyday beauty treatments.

Hair rinsing

After shampooing, rinse your hair with a 1 pint (500ml) jug of warm water to which you have added 2 tablespoons of cider vinegar. The vinegar rinse will remove any product build-up and make hair smooth and shiny.

Cleaning semi-permanent plaits, or dreadlocks
Fill a spray bottle with 1 part cider vinegar and 4 parts water. Spray plaits or dreadlocks generously, leave for 10 minutes, then rinse well. This helps remove grease and hair products such as wax.

Mouthwash
Minerals found in cider vinegar (such as potassium, sodium, copper and calcium) support oral health and cider vinegar is a traditional remedy for bad breath. Add a teaspoon of cider vinegar to a cup of warm water and gargle with the mixture, making sure to spit it out afterwards.

Chip-free nail polish
Apply cider vinegar to finger nails on a cotton wool ball and leave to dry before painting on nail polish – some people swear that it helps to make polish stay chip-free for longer.

Razor rash
The exfoliating properties in cider vinegar make it an ideal treatment for ingrown hairs. Apply a small amount of vinegar on a cotton wall ball to the affected area – the vinegar will help to remove dead skin cells.

Clearing blackheads
Twice a day, clean and dry your face. In a small bowl, mix 1 tablespoon of baking soda (bicarbonate of soda) with about 1 teaspoon of water to make a paste. Rub this over your skin to help loosen and remove blackheads, leave for 10–20 minutes, then rinse. Now help to restore your skin's natural acidity by patting on a little cider vinegar (apple cider vinegar).

Deodorizing
Wash your armpits, and then apply either neat cider vinegar, or cider vinegar in which you have steeped some rosemary or mint leaves, or lavender flowers, for 2 weeks.

Foot soak
Wash your feet, then soak them for 5–10 minutes in a basin of warm water containing half a cup of cider vinegar. This DIY spa treatment will help to treat foot odour, cracked heals, hard skin and fungal infections.

Not all cider vinegars available in stores are of the same quality. Refer to the guidelines on pages 10–11 when choosing vinegar to use in natural beauty treatments, or even better, make your own (see pages 11–12).

Skin cleansing and toning
Cider vinegar is perfect for maintaining the skin's natural acidity (for more on this, see page 85), whether combined with other natural ingredients, or just diluted with water. It is not recommended to apply neat vinegar to the skin, as it may be too acidic.

Cleansing oatmeal scrub

½ cup oatmeal   cider vinegar

1   Put the oatmeal into a small bowl, and add enough cider
    vinegar to moisten.
2   Rub the mixture into the skin, and then rinse off with warm
    water.

Use a larger quantity of oatmeal if you want to cleanse your whole
body this way.

Drinking cider vinegar diluted with water, or adding it to your diet in other ways is said to help to detox your liver and improve circulation. Improved circulation will make your skin look more glowing and healthy, and may also help to banish cellulite. For easy ways to add cider vinegar to your daily diet, see pages 21–32.

Vinegar bath

Put a cup of cider vinegar in the bath water, immerse a flannel (wash-cloth) in the water and use it to cleanse your skin.

Perfumes with apple notes are very popular – apple is one of the most-loved natural fragrances along with citrus, rose and vanilla. Apple scents work most obviously to impart a fresh summertime aroma for day-to-day wear, but autumnal scents more suited to evening wear are also available.

Skin rinsing

Wash in a shower or unplugged bath and rinse yourself with water. Then fill the bath with water, add half a cup of cider vinegar, lie in the bath and relax.

Alternatively, wash in the bath or shower. Then rinse yourself with warm water and half a cup of cider vinegar poured from a large plastic jug.

Skin toning

If you usually use cleansing cream or lotion on your face, follow this by applying a skin toner made by adding 4 tablespoons of cider vinegar to half a pint (250ml) of cold water. Keep the skin toner in a capped glass or plastic bottle, and apply it with a soft cotton cloth or cotton wool.

Scented toner

4 tablespoons cider vinegar
250ml (1 cup) cold water

½ tablespoon dried rosemary leaves or lavender flowers, or 1 tablespoon fresh leaves or flowers

1   Put the water and vinegar in a small pan over a medium heat.
2   Add the fresh or dried leaves or flowers and bring to the boil.
3   Simmer the mixture for 5 minutes, then allow to cool before transferring to a bottle.
4   Apply the toner to the skin with a soft cotton cloth or cotton wool.

> The anti-fungal and antibacterial properties in cider vinegar make it a real hero ingredient when it comes to fighting acne. Use it in treatments to remove excess oil from the skin, kill bacteria, clear black heads, and calm inflamed areas.

DIY vinegar face masks

Raid your fridge and kitchen cupboards to create these all-natural nourishing face masks – guaranteed to be kind and gentle on your skin.

Brightening face mask

1 teaspoon cider vinegar   1 tablespoon honey
1 teaspoon olive oil

1   Mix the ingredients in a small bowl until thoroughly combined.
2   Gently apply to the skin using your fingertips.
3   Relax for 15 minutes, then rinse off with warm water.

Pore-shrinking face mask

1 tablespoon cider vinegar   2 tablespoons sour cream

2 tablespoons honey

1   Mix the ingredients in a small bowl until thoroughly combined.

2   Gently apply to cleansed skin using your fingertips.

3   Relax for 15 minutes, then rinse off with cool water.

Exfoliating baking soda face mask

½ cup baking soda (bicarbonate
   of soda)
1 tablespoon apple cider
   vinegar

1 teaspoon lemon juice

1   Mix the ingredients together in a small bowl to form a paste.
2   Apply to clean skin in circular motions using your fingertips.
3   Sit for at least 10 minutes and then rinse off with warm water.

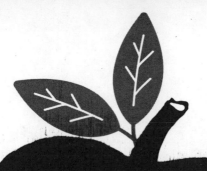

CHAPTER FIVE

NATURAL CLEANING PRODUCTS

NATURAL CLEANING PRODUCTS

Cider vinegar can make household chores easier and save the expense of buying household products. Making your own cleaning products may seem like a lot of work, but many of the suggestions in this chapter are extremely quick and easy, and use everyday ingredients that you will most likely find you already have in your storecupboard.

Making your own products is fun, and quite addictive. It will allow you to take control over your own environment, as well as saving you money. We all have busy lives, and it may seem easier to pick up a different brightly-coloured bottle for each of your household chores, but consider the benefits of leaving them behind in the store.

Greater control

Store-bought products often contain a cocktail of harsh chemicals which can be absorbed into the skin and breathed in. By making your own products you can be sure that only safe, natural ingredients are being used. You can also control the strength of the product by diluting as required, meaning that you can use the same product at different strengths for different tasks around the home.

More cost effective

Many of the ingredients used in natural cleaning products are easily available and inexpensive. The most commonly used ingredients storecupboard staples like lemons, vinegar and baking soda (bicarbonate of soda).

Environmentally friendly

The use of natural products is often referred to as 'green cleaning'. Making your own products cuts out the levels of pollution that are made during the production of commercial cleaning products, as well as reducing plastic consumption. Not all of the packaging for store-bought cleaning products is recyclable. Some commercial cleaning products may contain ingredients that are tested on animals.

Safer for pets and children

If you know that there are no 'nasties' in your cleaning products, you do not need to worry so much about other family members – especially pets and children – accidentally coming into contact with them. This also applies to any family members who might suffer from allergies – homemade natural products are unlikely to cause asthma attacks or irritation to the skin and eyes.

Create a nicer atmosphere

Homemade products that contain essential oils may have additional beneficial effects on your mood. Think of it as combining a deep cleaning session with an aromatherapy treatment for the whole family!

Using cider vinegar in natural cleaning products

Vinegar is one of the most effective naturally produced cleaning agents and can be used for a variety of tasks around the home. It is a mild acid, a corrosive and has antibacterial properties.

White vinegar is often used for household chores, but cider vinegar offers the same benefits and has a much more appealing scent. Like all vinegars, cider vinegar has antimicrobial properties and contains no hidden nasties. It makes a fantastic non-toxic cleaning product.

- Before cleaning any area with your homemade cider vinegar products, test a small area first.

Air-freshening

The smell of cider vinegar may not seem immediately appealing, but it is very effective at getting rid of strong unpleasant odours.

Room spray

Use as an air freshener to help eliminate the smell of smoke, pets, cooking and other unwanted odours.

1 teaspoon baking soda (bicarbonate of soda)

1 tablespoon cider vinegar

1   Half fill a spray bottle with water and add the baking soda (sodium bicarbonate) and cider vinegar.
2   Shake the open bottle to mix the contents.
3   When the foaming stops, fill the bottle up to the top with water and put on the cap.

Fragrant freshener

2 tablespoons cider vinegar

50g (2oz) fresh, or 25g (1oz) dried, lavender, thyme, rosemary or cloves

1   Add 2 pints (4¼ cups) water to a large saucepan and add the vinegar and fresh or dried herbs.
2   Mix well, place over a medium heat and bring to the boil.
3   Simmer for 10 minutes, then remove from the heat and allow to cool completely.
4   Strain the mixture, pour into a spray bottle and use as desired.

Kitchen smells
Add a splash of cider vinegar to soapy water then use this to wipe kitchen worktops or other hard surfaces to rid them of food smells or other unwanted odours.

Decorating odours
When painting a room, reduce strong paint smells by standing a bowl of cider vinegar somewhere safe.

Cleaning
The antibacterial and deodorizing properties of cider vinegar make it the perfect household cleaner.

Post-cooking cleanser
Rid your hands of the smell of onions, garlic or fish by pouring cider vinegar into your cupped hand, rubbing them together, and washing with soapy water.

Kitchen aid
Freshen and clean floors by adding a cup of cider vinegar to the cleaning water.

Help to keep sink and basin drains clear by pouring half a cup of baking soda (sodium bicarbonate) down the plughole, then half a cup of hot cider vinegar (heated for a minute in the microwave). Leave for half an hour and then flush with a kettle of just-boiled water.

Add half a cup of cider vinegar to dish-washing water to cut grease and reduce the amount of washing-up liquid that is needed.

Disinfecting

Immerse a smelly flannel, sponge or dishcloth in half and half of cider vinegar and water. Leave for two hours and then rinse with water.

Help prevent mould discolouring bathroom tile grout by spraying tiles twice a week with water containing two tablespoons of cider vinegar.

Clean a mildewed shower curtain by putting it in the washing machine along with a large bath towel. Before you start, add 4oz (100g) bicarbonate of soda to the washing powder in the dispenser. Then wash the load on a low-temperature setting, adding 100ml cider vinegar to the fabric-softener dispenser during the rinse cycle.

Fragrant bathroom cleaner

½ cup cider vinegar

3–4 drops eucalyptus or lavender essential oil

1   Mix the vinegar with an equal amount of water in a small bowl.
2   Add the essential oil and mix well.

Use the mixture to remove mildew and other stains from bathroom surfaces. For really stubborn stains, for example on baths or around taps, you may need to add more vinegar and less water.

Dishwasher care

Clean a smelly dishwasher or its dispenser with a brush and soapy water, then add a cup of cider vinegar to the empty machine and run a cycle to remove odours.

Glass cleaning

Wipe window glass, spectacle lenses, or mirrors with a mixture of 1 part cider vinegar to 3 parts water, then dry with newspaper or a slightly damp towel.

Limescale removing

Soften limescale around taps by covering overnight with a paper towel soaked in cider vinegar; next morning the limescale should be much easier to remove.

Help clear limescale from a steam-iron's reservoir by filling it with cider vinegar. Turn on the iron, let it steam until dry, then rinse the reservoir with clean water.

Polishing

Shine up wooden furniture by adding a few drops of cider vinegar to commercial polish.

Polish wooden furniture with half and half cider vinegar and paraffin.

Brighten copper and brass by applying a paste made of equal parts of salt, flour and cider vinegar. Let the paste dry for 10 minutes, then buff with a polishing cloth.

Rust removing

Help remove rust by immersing small metal objects in cider vinegar for several hours.

Stain removing

Wipe salt-stained shoes with a cup of water containing a tablespoon of cider vinegar.

Clean stained stainless-steel, or copper-coated pans and bowls with a paste of salt and cider vinegar.

Try removing ink, grass, coffee, tea, fruit and berry stains from fabric by soaking the stain in cider vinegar for an hour, then washing.

Clean brown stains inside a tea or coffee pot by filling it with half and half cider vinegar and water. Leave for half an hour then rinse.

Sticky-stuff remover

Loosen stickers or remnants of their glue by gently scrubbing with cider vinegar.

Use cider vinegar to remove the resin and hardener components of two-part epoxy glue, or even not-yet-set glue. (If any of these touch your eye or skin, irrigate the area immediately and generously with water).

Loosen chewing gum or its stains on clothes by rubbing with cider vinegar before laundering.

Devices

Wipe down digital devices such as smart phones, tablets and computer keyboards with a little cider vinegar on a damp cloth – this will remove germs and make them shiny as new.

Sink pipes

Help clear a blockage by pouring 200g/7oz/1 cup baking soda (bicarbonate of soda) down the plughole, followed by

240ml/8fl oz/1 cup hot cider vinegar. Wait for 30 minutes, then flush with a kettle of just-boiled water. If necessary, use a sink plunger.

Garden and grace

As well as being an invaluable help around the house, cider vinegar can also prove useful in the garden and for car maintenance.

Insect repelling

Repel fleas by adding half a cup of cider vinegar to the final rinsing water when shampooing your dog.

Weedkilling

Kill weeds by spraying with cider vinegar.

Windscreen anti-icer

Mix 3 parts cider vinegar with 1 part water and use this to wipe over your windscreen.

Laundry

It is definitely worth keeping a bottle of cider vinegar in your laundry room to help with stubborn stains, smells and scaling.

Fabric softener

2 tablespoons cider vinegar
2 tablespoons baking soda
(bicarbonate of soda)

1   Add 4 tablespoons cold water to a small jar or bowl.
2   Mix in the cider vinegar and baking powder (bicarbonate
    of soda).
3   Add the mixture to the final rinse water if washing by hand, or
    to the fabric-softener dispenser of a washing machine, to leave
    fabrics soft and static-free.

Stain remover
Rub soiled collars and cuffs with a paste of equal parts of
cider vinegar and baking soda (sodium bicarbonate). Wait
for 30 minutes then wash as normal.

Reduce perspiration stains on clothing by soaking
garments for several hours in a basin of water containing
half a cup of cider vinegar.

Colour setting
When washing coloured fabric add a cup of cider vinegar to
help set the dye so it won't leach out and stain other fabrics.

Tights
Make tights longer-lasting and less ladder-prone by adding
a tablespoon of cider vinegar to the final rinse water when
washing.

Washing machine care

If your washing machine or its dispenser is smelly, clean with a brush and soapy water, then add a cup of cider vinegar to the empty machine and run a cycle to remove the odour.

If your washing-machine dispenser is furred up with lime-scale, clean with a brush and soapy water, then add a cup of cider vinegar to the dispenser and run a cycle to help remove the deposits.

INDEX